YOUR KNOWLEDGE HAS VALUE

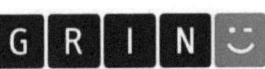

Anti-Helminthic and Pesticidal Effect of Heliotropium Indicum Linn. Pharmacology of Natural Products

Asamoah Larbi

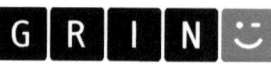

Bibliographic information published by the German National Library:

The German National Library lists this publication in the National Bibliography; detailed bibliographic data are available on the Internet at http://dnb.dnb.de.

ISBN: 9783346626790
This book is also available as an ebook.

© GRIN Publishing GmbH
Nymphenburger Straße 86
80636 München

Print and binding: Books on Demand GmbH, Norderstedt, Germany
Printed on acid-free paper from responsible sources.

The present work has been carefully prepared. Nevertheless, authors and publishers do not incur liability for the correctness of information, notes, links and advice as well as any printing errors.

GRIN web shop: https://www.grin.com/document/1188315

UNIVERSITY OF CAPE COAST

SCHOOL OF PHYSICAL SCIENCES

DEPARTMENT OF LABORATORY TECHNOLOGY

ANTI-HELMINTHIC AND PECTICIDAL EFFECTS OF *HELIOTROPIUM INDICUM LINN*

BY

ASAMOAH LARBI

A DISSERTATION PRESENTED TO THE DEPARTMENT OF LABORATORY TECHNOLOGY, UNIVERSITY OF CAPE COAST IN PARTIAL FULFILMENT OF THE REQUIREMENTS FOR THE AWARD OF B.SC. LABORATORY TECHNOLOGY DEGREE.

2013

ABSTRACT

This work evaluates the aqueous extract of inflorescences, leaves and roots of *Hetropium inddicum linn* for its anti-helminthic and insecticidal properties. The extracts were prepared using Asumeng's protocol (Asumeng, et al, 2012). The prepared crude extracts were subjected to photochemical screening using standard techniques of plant secondary metabolites. The extracts were tested for alkaloid, flavonoids, saponins, tannins, Anthraquinones, reducing sugars (in glycosides) cardiac glycosides, and glycosides. Evaluation of anti-helminthic effect of the plant extracts showed that, although all the three screened plant extracts exhibit anti-helminthic activity, the leaf extract appears to have high anti-helminthic effect than the inflorescence and the root extracts. The inflorescence extract had more anti-helminthic activity than the root extract and this activity increases as concentration increases for each extract. It was also found from the results that the extracts have no effect on the weevil (*Sitophilus Zeamais*).

TABLE OF CONTENTS

CHAPTER ONE: INTRODUCTION

1.1 Background

Herbalism or herbal medicine has long tradition of use outside conventional medicine. It is emerging as a mainstream medicinal intervention as improvement in quality control analysis and quality assurance systems along with advance clinical research show the value of herbal medicine in treating and preventing diseases. Herbal medicine is also called botanical medicine or phytomedicine, it has been defined by several research and academic scholars, however it is basically referred to as the use of plant parts such as seed, berries roots, leaves, back, or flowers (inflorescences) for medicinal purpose (Ehrlich, 2011).

The importance of medicinal plants in the prevention and the treatment of diseases cannot be underscored. For instance, most medicinal plants serve as sources of *lead compounds* in the synthesis of potent drugs such as anti-heminthics agent. The importance if further enhanced due to the fact that cost and accessibility of orthodox drugs that are used in the treatment of diseases including helminthiases, makes it difficult for most people to adapt thereby making search for alternative ones with lower cost and more accessible inevitable (Marcus, 2009).

Several clinical symptoms such as irritation, discomfort, malfunction of organs or the overall breakdown of the body system indicates diseases conditions which may lead to permanent disability or death of the host or patient. Considering the effects of disease conditions on people and the economic importance of these citizens in increasing nation's wealth or national development, alternative medicine therefore becomes an important therapeutic practice, technique and belief outside the practice of mainstream Western healthcare with equal or high clinical importance at low economic value or cost. For example, alternative medicine enhances therapies that improve quality life, prevent diseases and address conditions that conventional medicine may have limited success in curing, including helminthiasis and may also have pesticidal properties that will be more useful for pest control application as part of agricultural pest management methods with no chemical residue (Wright et al 2007).

1.2 Statement of problem

Helminthic infection

One major problem in West Africa today is worm infestation. According to WHO (2007) worm infestation is a common reason for seeking medical help in various African countries particularly Ghana, with up to 4.9% of hospital admission in some areas resulting from the complication of

1

intestinal worm infections and as many as 3% of hospitalizations are attributable to ascariasis alone. However, recommended drugs for the treatment of the above infection are expensive and not assessable to the vulnerable or average citizen, thus making it difficult for most people, especially those in rural areas to come by of adopt.

Insect infestation

Farmers are saddled with several challenges which include low soil fertility, pest infestations, and other diseases conditions in plant or crops. The most alarming problem in grain production is insect infestation (grain weevils) resulting in destruction of stored grains by farmers in most villages. Consequently, income level has drastically reduced leading to low standard of living in most grain producing villages in Ghana, food insecurity and increase in in rural unemployment. Chemicals that are used in the control of these food pests are very expensive and complex in most farmers and also raises pesticide residue concerns for grain consumers.

1.3 Justification

Wold Health Organization (WHO) intestinal helminthes treatment guide, suggest that one popular approach for the control of worm infection is by deworming (WHO, 2007). Review of treatments of worm infestation have shown that WHO's recommendation well adhered to, however most of these deworming drugs administered by clinicians are solely orthodox such as *albendazole* and *mebendazole*. The adoption of orthodox drugs such as albendazole and mobendazole alone for clinical treatment suggest potential treatment difficulty of worm infestation in rural communities due to high cost and lack of accessibility and availability, and thus call for alternative medicine with high potency and low cost to argument the existing orthodox drugs and increase accessibility and availability of deworming drugs at low cost.

1.4 Hypothesis

The inflorescences, leaves and roots of *hliotropium indicum linn* have no significant ant-helmenthic and pesticidal properties

1.5. Aim

The aim of this study was to evaluate the aqueous extract of inflorescences, leaves and roots of *hliotropium indicum linn* for its no significant ant-helmenthic and pesticidal properties.

2

1.6 Objectives

The objective of this research were:

1.6.1 To determine the mean time of paralysis of helminthes and grain weevil in aqueous extract of inflorescences, leaves and roots of *hliotropium indicum linn.*

1.6.2 To determine the mean time of death of helminthes and grain in aqueous extract of inflorescences, leaves and roots of *hliotropium indicum linn.*

CHAPTER TWO: LITERATURE REVIEW

2.1 Herbal medicine

Herbal medicine has its root in prehistory making every bit as ancient tradition as farming or cooking. In the Graeco-Roman era, Hippocrates (father medicine), theophratus (father of botany), Galen (originator of pharmaceutical galenicals) and Dioscoroides were all herbalists (Moody, 2007). Also about one-quarter of the prescription drugs dispensed by community pharmacy in the United States contain at least one active ingredient derived from plants (Farnsworth and Morries, 1992). Also in Ghana, around 205 medicinal plant species are very common in nature in the Northern, Western, Central and Eastern zones of the country (FEPA, 1992). Beyond the problem of trying to test herbal preparations that may contain active ingredients in the question of whether the research eventually will lead to the isolation of single active ingredient that can be packaged and sold.

Intense debate surrounds the issue of how to conduct clinical trials of herbal medicine according to the Western Pharmaceutical Clinical Standards. Critics however says there is an inherent problem with the single active ingredient approach preferred by pharmaceutical companies that are actively involved in herbal medicine research. It is argued that isolating a single compound may not be the most appropriate approach preferred in situations where a plant's activity decreases on further fractionation (separation of active ingredients by using solvents) or where the plants contain two or three active ingredients that must be taken together to produce the full effect (Chaudhurry, 1992). Beckstrom-Sternber & Duke (1994) have documented several cases where synergy has been lost by using the single ingredient approach to developing drugs from plants.

The public pay high prices for orthodox medicine because the cost for experimental techniques through Research and Development (R and D) is enormous. Another common perception is that orthodox medicine which is scientifically based is more reliable, safer and more effective. This

3

notion may be wrong because drugs once thought to be safe are often withdrawn from the market for causing severe side effects and even fatalities. The thalidomide fiasco for early morning sickness gave birth to deformed babies. Again, antibiotics which created false hope that modern medical science could eradicate diseases caused by body's resistance to harmful bacteria (Bradstreet, 1998). Recently, in Nigeria, the National Agency for Food and Drug Administration and Control (NAFDAC) banned the use of Novalgin (a potent analgesic and antipyretic agent) because of its severe side effects that led to the death of children (Osemene et al, 2011).

Although, the history of orthodox medicine traces its root back to Hippocrates, the father of medicine, the practice of orthodox medicine today is not strictly in line with the principles of fathers of medicine (Rees and Shuter, 1996).

Orthodox medicine began over a century ago during the period of Renaissance. As at then the objective thinking of the causative theory of modern science replaced the ecological model which had predominated for over 2000 years (Bhikha, 2004). The new paradigm is often termed the Cartesian model being named after the French philosopher, Rene Descartes (1596-1650). This model, it was claimed, invalidated the humoral concepts of the holistic principles of Hippocrates. Galen and Ibn Sina promoted the ideology that man was separated from nature could be viewed objectively through experiment (Boussel et al, 1982). This heralded the birth of scientific or orthodox medicine. The frontiers of orthodox medicine were further broadened by Rudolph Virdow (1821-1902) who demonstrated that disease begins with changes in living cells and by Louis Pasteur (1822-1895) whose role in the development of germ theory of infection was key importance (Ree & Shuter, 1996; Gilbert et al, 1998); Bhikha & Haq, 2000).

Under the germ theory, disease was associated with specific micro-organisms. Since, then technology through research and development (R and D) had played tremendous roles in the propagation of orthodox medicine which is scientifically based and evolve along certain specifications or routes. These routes led to the manifestations of plethora of specialists in disorders of specific organs, tissue and cells such as cardiologists, dermatologists and neurologists among others. Hence it has been advocated that patients should be regarded as collections of separate body parts and organ systems (Thomas, 2002). Generally, the philosophy of orthodox medicine is exclusively based on the physical world and excludes any explanation that goes beyond this (Hummond-Tooke, 1989; Gilbert et al, 1998). For instance, health and illness are seen as a relationship between the body's components and sub-structure while the mind is considered

4

independent of the body. The causes of disease are therefore scientific and presented in terms of such concepts as chemical imbalance, virus replication, serum level overload and so on (Bhikha, 2004).

Technology based scientific research in herbal medicine perhaps has made some significant impact in addressing some prominent doubts about herbal preparations such as packaging problems, level of hygiene and dosage regimen. Presently, most herbal medicine sold in Ghana come with well specified dosage regimen, packaged in pharmaceutically approved forms such as ointments, creams, tablets, capsules and coloured but flavoured syrups (Sampson, 1995). However, unlike orthodox medicines, no injectable form of herbal medicine is available in Africa. Furthermore, there has been marked improvement in the packaging of most herbal medicines. Also, the rate of advertisement of herbal medicines in both the print and electronic media is high and unrestricted unlike for orthodox medicines where some *Over The Counter (OTC)* drugs are advertised especially if they are listed or registered with regulatory bodies Food and drug authorities (Osemene et al, 2011).

Also, plants have been used for medicinal purpose long before recorded history. Ancient Chinese and Egyptian papyrus writings describe medicinal uses for plants as early as 3000BC. Indigenous culture (such as African and Native American) used herbs in their healing rituals, whiles others developed traditional medicine systems (such as Ayundrveda and traditional Chinese medicine) in which verbal therapies were used. Researchers found that people in different parts of the world tended to use the same or similar plant for the same purpose (Blackman et al, 2009). It also indicated that, in the early 19th century, when chemical analysis first became available, scientists began to extract and modify the active ingredients from plants. Later, chemists began making their own version of plant compounds, and over time, the use of herbal medicines declined in favour of drugs (Dabidian et al, 2007). Almost one fourth of pharmaceutical drugs and derived from botanicals. Most research has been conducted by some great researchers and research institutions, confirming that natural/herbal drugs be used over orthodox drugs (Bradstreet et al, 1998; Mood, 2007).

Recently, the world health organization estimated that about 80% of people worldwide rely on herbal medicine for some part of their primary health care (WHO,2007). In Germany, about 600-700 plant based medicines are available and are prescribed by some 70% of German physician. In the past 20 years in the United States, public dissatisfaction with the cost of prescription medications, combined with an interest in returning to natural or herbal organic remedies, has led

5

to an increase in herbal medicine used. The used of herbal supplement has increased dramatically over the past 30 years. Herbal supplements are classified as dietary supplements by US Dietary Supplement Health and Education Act (DSHEA) of 1994. That means herbal supplements unlike prescription drugs can be sold without being tested to approve they are safe and effective. However, herbal supplements must be made according to good manufacturing and practices (Sood et al, 2007).

Studies shows that nearly one-third of Americans use herbs. Unfortunately, a study in *New England Journal of Medicine* found that nearly 70% of people taking herbal medicine (most of whom were well educated and had a high than average income) were reluctant to tell their doctors that they used complementary and alternative medicine (Osemene, et al, 2011). Statistics has shown that the use of drugs is on a very high increase in both advanced and developing countries (Osemene et al, 2011).

2.2 Heliotropium Indicum Linn Plant

2.2.1 Anatomy

Heliotropium indicum Linn is an annual, erect, branched, hirsute plant; 15 to 50 centimeters high. Leaves are opposite or alternate, ovate to oblong-ovate, somewhat hairy, acute or acuminate, base decurrent along the petiole, 3 to 8 centimeters long. Flowers are small, and borne on one side of curved, terminal, or leaf-opposed spikes which are 3 to 8 centimeters long. Carlyx is green. Corolla is pale lavender to nearly white, funnel-shaped, and about 5 millimeters long, with a slender and cylinderic tube and the limb 3 to 3.5 millimeters in diameter. Samens are 5, inserted on the corolla tube. Ovary completely or imperfectly 4-called, 4 ovules style terminal or leave opposed, 3 to 10cm long, flowers all in one side, the lower ones opening first. Fruit is 4-5 millimeters long, composed of 2 ovoid, beaked nutlets (Reddy et al, 2002).

2.2.2. Uses

Heliotropium indicum Linn as a medicinal plant is widely used in West Africa, India and the Philippians. It is used extensively among rural dwellers and some urban dwellers in Ghana (Ainsle, 1937). Its leaves have traditionally been used in medicine abortifacients, ecobolics, antidotes (venomous stings, bites), anti-arthritics, eye treatments, febrifuges, analgesics, and vermifuges. It has been used in managing epilepsy and convulsion. The whole plant has activity against diarrhea, dysentery, tumours and cancers (Burkill, 1935, Dalziel, 1937, Quisumbing *et at, 1957;* Oliver, 1960, Irvine, 1961 and Kugelman, 1976).

6

2.2.3. Uses

Heliotropium indicum Linn as a medical plant is widely used in West Africa, India and Philippines. It is extensively among rural dwellers and some urban dwellers in Ghana (Ainsle, 1927). Its leaves have traditionally been used in medicine abortifacients, ecoboplics, antidotes (venomous sting, bites), anti-arthritics, eye treatments, febrifuges, analgesics, vermifuges. It has been used in managing epilepsy and convulsion. The whole plant has activity against diarrhea, dysentery, tumours and cancers (Burkill, 1935; Dalziel, 1937; Quisumbing et al, 1957; Oliver, 1960; Irvine, 1961 and Kugelman, 1976).

Gastroprotective/antimicrobial use: Studies have shown that aqueous extract of dried leaves of *Heliotropium indicum Linn* have dose-dependent gastroprotective effects. For instance, a wound healing study of 10% topical application increase the percentage of wond contraction, increase tonsil strength and decrease time of healing from rapid epithelization and collagenisation. Another study showed that ethanolic extract of the plant showed better wound healing activity than *P zeylanicum* and *A indica*. Other studies showed significant promotion of wound healing with methanol and aqueous extracts. In the wound infection model (*Stapp aureus and P. aeruginosa*), the methanol extract showed significant healing activity compared to standard *nitrofurazone* (Adelaja, et al, 2008).

Anti-tumor use: studies have again revealed that isolated oxide of alkaloid indicine from the plant showed significant anti-tumor activity in *carcinosarcoma, leaukemia,* and *melanoma tumor* systems. Additionally, anti-inflammatory study of *H indicum* produced significant anti-inflammatory effect in both acute and subacute models of inflammation, with activities comparable to *acetylsalicylic acid* and *phenylbutazone* respectively. Other studies also showed that petroleum and ethanol extracts exhibited considerable anti-inflammatory activity compared with ketorolac trimethamine as standard (Srinivas, 2000).

Anti-tuberculosis use: study on volatile oil from the aerial parts of the plant of the plant showed significant antituberculosis activity against *M tuberculosis*. The major constituents were phytol, e-dodecanol, and B-linalool. Anti-tumor study on extracts of the plant yielded an active principle, an *N-oxide* of the alkaloid indcine, which showed significant activity in several experimental tumor systems (Lloydia, 1976).

2.2.4. Studies

So many studies have been carried out on the plant which includes: Gastroprotective/Antimicrobial (Study of the aqueous extracts of dried leaves of Heliotropium indicum showed dose-dependent

7

gastroprotective effects) Wound healing ((1) study of 10% topical application increased the percentage of wound contraction, increased tensile strength and decreased time of healing from rapid epithelization and collagenisation. (2) Ethanolic extract of the plant showed better wound healing with methanol and aqueous extracts. In the wound infection model (Staph aureus and P. aeruginosa), the methanol extract showed significant healing activity compared to standard nitrofurazone). (Adelaja et al, 2008).

Anti-Tumor (Isolated oxide of alkaloid indicine from the plant showed significant anti-tumor activity in carcinosarcoma, leukaemia, and melanoma tumor systems), and Anti-Inflammatory ((1) Study of H indicum produced significant anti-inflammatory effect in both acute and subacute models of inflammation, with activities comparable to acetylsalicclic acid and phenylbutazone respectively. (2) Petroleum and ethanol extracts exhibited considerable anti-inflammatory activity compared with ketorolac trimethamine as standard). (Srinivas, 2000).

Anti-Tuberculosis (Study of the volatile oil from the aerial parts of the plant showed significant anti-tuberculosis activity against M tuberculosis. The major constituents were phytol, e-dodecanol, and β-linalool), Anti-Tumor (extract study yielded an active principle, an Oxide of the alkaloid indicine, which showed significant activity in several experimental tumor systems). (Lloydia, 1976).

Immunostimulant Effect: Dried leaves extract significantly increased in vito phagocytic index and lymphycocyte viability in all assys, increase in antibody titer and delayed-type hypersebsitivity in mice. Results conclude a dose-dependent immunostimulant effect, probably due to the alkaloid content or combination of other components. A pastroprotective effect. Phytochemical analysis yielded alkaloid, saponins and tennins. A gastroprotyective function is through its ability to mobilize endogenouse prostaglandins in the gastric mucosa), etc. (Lloydia, 1976 and Reddy et al, 2002).

2.3. Worm infection

Parasitic worms, often referred to as helminths are division of eukaryotic parasites. They are worm-like organisms living in and feeding on living hosts' nutrients absorption, causing weakness and disease. those that live inside the digestive tract are called intestinal parasites. They can live inside humans and other animals. Montresor et al. (2002).

8

2.3.1. intestinal helminths

Intestinal helminths are types of intestinal parasites that reside in the human gastrointestinal tract (Pollitt *et al*, 1997). They represent one of the most prevalent forms of parasitic tract disease. Scholars estimate that over a quarter of the world's population is infected with an intestinal worm of some sort, with roundworm, hookworm and whipworm infecting 1.47 billion people, 1.05 billion people, and 1.30 billion people respectively. Furthermore, the world bank estimates that 100 million people may experience stunting or wasting as a result of infection. (Petri *et al*, 2006).

Because of their high mobility and lower standards of hygiene, school-age children are particularly vulnerable to these parasites (Montressor *et al*, 2002). Overall, it is estimated that 400 million, 170 million and 300 million children are infected with roundworm, hookworm and whipworm respectively. Children may also be particulary susceptible to the adverse effects of helminth infections due to their incomplete physical development and their greater immunological vulnerability. Boivin *et al*, (1993) and Amara E. *et al*, (2005).

2.3.2. Categorization

Parasitic wprms belongs to four groups: monogeneans, cestodes (tapeworms), nematodes (roundworms), and trematodes (flukes). The following table shows the principal morphological distinctions for each of these helminth families (Petri *et al*, (2006):

TABLE 2.1. A table showing principal morphological distinctions for helminth families

	Cestodes (tapeworms)	Trematodes (flukes)	Nematodes (Roundworms)
Shades	Segmented plane	Unsegmented plane	Cylindrical
Body cavity	No	No	Present
Body covering	Tegument	Tegument	Cuticle
Digestive tube	No	Ends in cecum Hermaphroditic.	Ends in anus
Sex	Hermaphroditic	Except schistosomes which are dioecious	Dioecious
Attachment organs	Sucker or bothridia, and rostellum with hooks		

9

		Oral sucker and ventral sucker or acetabulum	Lips, teeth, filariform extremities, and dentary plates
	Tapeworm infection		
Example diseases in human		Schistosomiasis, swimmer's itch	Ascariasis, Dracunculiasis, elephantiasis, enterrobiasis (pinworm), filariasis, hookworm, onchocerciasis, trichinosis, trichuriasis (whipworm)

2.3.3. Acquision

Helminths often find their way into a host through contaminated food or water, soil, mosquitoe bites, and even sexual acts.poorly washed eaten raw may contain eggs of nematodes suc as Ascaris, *Enterobius, Thichuris,* and/or cestodes such as *taenia, hymenolepis,* and *Echinococus.* Plants may also be contaminated with flukes matacercaria (*e.g. Fasciola*). *Diphyllobothrium* (fish), and *Paragonimus* (crustaceans). Schistosomes and nematodes such as hookworms (*Ancylostoma* and *Necator*) and *Strongyloides* can penetrate the skin (Maizles, 2003). Finally, *Wuchereriar, Onchocerca,* and *Dracunculus* are transmitted by mosquitoes and flies.

Populations in the developing world are at particular risk for infestation parasitic worms (Levinger, 1992). Risk factors include inadequate water treatment, use of contaminated water for drinling, cooking, irrigation and to wash food, undercooked food of animal origin, and walking barefoot. Simple measures can have strong impacts on prevention. These include use of shoes, soaking vegetables with 1.5% bleach, adequate cooking of foods, and sleeping under mosquito-proof nets. Petri *et al,* (2006).

2.3.4. Immune Response

Response to worm ionfection in humans is a YTh2 (T helper cells, suv-group of lymphocutes) response in the majority of cases. Inflammation of the gut may also occure, resulting in cycst-like

10

structures forming around the egg deposits throughout the body. The host`s lymphatic system is also increasibgly taxed the longer helminths propagate, as they excrete toxins after feeding. These toxins are released into the intestines to be absorbed by the host`s bloodstream. This phenomenon makes the host susceptible to more common diseases, such as viral and bacterial infections. Maizels *et al,* (2003).

2.3.5. Costs of intestinal helminth infection

2.3.5.1. Symptoms

Patients with heavy worm loads, and parasitic infection are frequently symptomatic. Conditions associations with intestinal helminth infection include intestinal obstruction, insomnia, vomiting and weakness, and stomach pains; while the natural movement of worms and their attachment to the intestine may be generally uncomfortable for their hosts. The migration of Ascaris larva through the respiratory passageways can also lead to temporary asthma and other respiratory symptoms. Petri *et al,* (2006).

In addition to low-level cost of chronic infection, helminthic infection may be punctuated by the need for more serious, urgent care; for example, the World Health Organisation found that worm infection is common reason for seeking medical help in a variety of countries, with up to 4.9% of hospital admissions in some areas resulting from the complications of intestinal worm infection and as many as 3% of hospitalization attributable to ascariasis alone. (WHO, 1987).

The fact that immune response triggered by helminth infection may drain the body`s ability to fight other diseases, making the affected individuals more prone to co-infections. There are reasonable evidences indicating that helminthiasis is responsible for the unrelenting prevalence of AIDS and tuberculosis in developing countries, particularly African countries. Several data clearly reveal that effective treatment of helminth infection reduces human immune virus (HIV) progression and viral load, obviously by improving helminth-induce immune suppression. Bentwich *et al,* (2002).

2.3.5.2. Nutrition

One way in which the intestinal helminthes may inpair the development of their human hosts is through their impact on nutrition. Intestinal helminth infection has associated problems such as vitamin deficiencies, stunting, anaemia, and protein-energy malnutrition, which in turn affect cognitive ability and intellectual development. This relationship is particularly alarming because it is gradual and often relatively asymptomatic. Rebecca, *et al,* (2003) and Crompton, *et al,* (1993).

Parasite infection may affect nutrition in several ways. On the other hand, some scholars argue that worms may compete directly with their hosts for access to nutrients; both whipworm and

11

roundworm and believed to impact their hosts this way. Nonetheless, Watkins and Pollitt (Pollitt et al, 1997) argue that the magnitude of this effect is likely be minimal; after all, nutritional requirements of these intestinal worms are small when compared with that of their host organisms. A more probable source of infection-induced malnutrition is the nutrient malabsorption associated with parasite presence in the body. For example, in both pigs and humans, *Ascaries* has been tied to temporarily induced lactose intolerance and Vitamin A, nitrogen, and fat malabsorption. Impaired nutrient uptake may result from direct damage to intestine's mucosal walls as a result of worms' presence, but may be consequence of more nuanced changes such as chemical imbalance caused by body's reaction to the helminths. Alternatively, Wetkins and Pollitt (Pollitt et al, 1997) suggest that the worms 'release of protease inhibitors to defend against the body's digestive process may impair the breakdown of their nutritious substances as well. Levinger (1992) mentions this briefly in the case of whipworm. Finally, worm infections may also cause diarrhoea and speed "transit time" through the intestinal system, further reducing the body's opportunity to retain nutrients in food.

Worms may also contribute to malnutrition by creating anorexia. A decline in appetite and food consumption due to helminthic infection in widely recognised by literature, with a recent study of 459 children in Zanzibar reporting that even mother noticed spontaneous increase in appetite after their children underwent a deworming regime. Although the exact cause of such anorexia is not known, researchers believe that it may be a side effect of body's immune response to the worm and stress of combating infection. Specifically, some of the cytokines released in the immune response have been tied to anorexic reactions in animals. Crompton, et al, (1993).

Helminthes may also affect nutrition by inducing iron-deficiency anemia. This is most severe in heavy hookworm infections as *N. Americanus* and *A. Duodenale* feed directly on the blood of their host. Although the impact of individual worms is limited (each consumes about 0.02-0.07ml of blood daily, respectively) this may nonetheless add up in individuals with heavy infections, since they may carry hundreds of worms at a given time. one scholar went so far as to predict, "the blood loss caused by hookworm was equivalent to the daily exsanguination (process of blood loss, to a degree sufficient to cause death) of 1.5 million people", while a study in Zanzibar showed a 15¢triannual application of mebendazole could avert 0.251 of blood loss per child per year. (Petri et al, 2006). Although, whipworm is milder in its effects, it may also induce anaemia as a result of the bleeding caused by its damage to the small intestine. Crompton, et al, (1993).

The connection between worm burden and malnutrition is further supported by studies indicating deworming programs lead to sharp increases in growth; the presence of this result even in older children than was previously believed. "Walson et al, (2009).

2.3.5.3. Delayed intellectual development

Once the links between helminth infection and various forms of malnutrition are established, a number of pathways of parasite burden may affect cognition. For example, poor performance on normal growth indicators appears to be correlated with lower school performance on normal growth indicators appears to be correlated with lower school achievement and enrolment, worse results on some forms of testing, and a decreased ability tp focus; iron deficiency may result in "mild growth retardation", difficulty with abstract cognitive task, and "lower scores on tests of mental and motor development as well as increased fearfulness, inattentiveness, and decreased social responsiveness" among very young children, Anaemia has also been associated with reduced stamina for physical labour, a decline in the ability to learn new information, and "apathy, irritability, and fatigue" . Giordiani et al (1992).

These connections are supported by a number of deworming studies. For example, using 47 students from the Democratic Republic of Congo, iron suppliments acted as a complement to deworming medication, producing better effects on mental cognition when they were applied in conjunction than when they were individually administered.

This result may be because iron supplements may "improve (students`) physical wellbeing to the point of enhancing attentional or arousal mechanism influential in leaning and cognitive performance", with deworming medication only acting to extend these benefits by further reducing the tendency to anaemia. Nokes et al. (1992).

A number of papers take the study of intestinal helminth the malnutrition cognition link to focus on the connection between worm infections and memory formation. For example, interventions to reduce whipworm infection in 159 Jamaican schoolchildren led to better "auditory short-term memory" and "scanning and retrieval of long-term memory," particularly fascinating was his discovery that a nine-week period was all that was necessary for dewormed students to "catch up" to their worm-free peers in test performance. Nokes (Nokes et al. 1992) optimistic conclusion that "whipworm infection adverse effect on certain cognitive functions reversible by therapy" is particularly significant because it suggests the effects of worms on intellectual performance may not be restricted to the mechanism of long-term malnutrition, since the physical and developmental effects of such malnutrition would theoretically be irreversible.

13

Ezeamama *et al.* (2005) and Sakti *et al.* (1999) studied worm burden in the Phillipians and Indonesia, respectively. Both authors found significant negative impcacts of helminthic infection on memory and fluency, findings that are particularly meaningful because they are included controls for socioeconomic status, haemoglobin level, and proxies of nutrition (nutritional status and stunting, respectively), as Ezaemama observes, these studies suggest "undernutrition is not the primary mediator of the observed relationships" between worm infection and intellectual performance, particularly because their findings were significant in aspects of intellect that went beyond more cognition and reaction time.

Finally, much as physical activity of nutritionally mediated patients with heavy worm burden struggle to preserve energy and fight malnutrition, so too could the poorly nourished mind similarly adapt by reducing mental effort in the form of arousal and sustained attention. While they find little evidence this adaptation would provide benefits in the form of energy conservation, the active course of ongoing parasitic disease clearly imposes other, more limitation on an individual's attention span. Nokes *et al.* (1992) and Sakti *et al.* (1999).

2.3.5.4. Schools attendance and outcomes

the day-to-day costs of illness provide a strong explanation for yet another negative consequence of helminth infection, or the observation that acts as a very real barrier to children`s progress in school as quantified by outcome measure measures such as absenteeism, under-enrolment, and attrition. Students may be too weak to attend classes, or their school enrolment fees. This effect may be conceptually distinct from previous findings about the impact of parasitism on cognition and learning; for example, deworming programs improve school attendance by 25% without affecting test outcomes at all. Nonetheless, these effects may also be related; school attendance and enrolment grew significantly in the school-age populations that benefited most from the Rockefeller Foundation`s deworming programs, leading to a long-term increase in income, as well as a rise in literacy rates. Marek *et al,* (1996), Montressor *et al,* (2002) and Nokes *et at,* (1992)

CHAPTER THREE: MATERIALS AND METHODS

3.1. Plant Sample Collection and Authentication

The plant was collected in Amamoma, Cape Coast-Ghana and authenticated at the herbarium of school of Biological Sciences, University of Cape Coast.

3.2. Parasite Collection

20 helminthes were collected from the Cape Coast abattoir

20 grain weevils were collected from Agric Village maize deport U.C.C.

3.3. Preparation of Plant Extracts (Asumeng *et al,* 2012)

The various parts of *Heliotropium Indicum Linn* were air dried for 8 days under shade and powdered using laboratory mill at Organic Chemistry Laboratory of University of Cape Coast.300g of each powder was soaked in 150ml of distilled water, shaken for 15 minutes and then heated for about 25 minutes in a hot bath. It was allowed to cool and then filtered. The filtrate was concentrated by evaporation over a hot water bath and hot air given at 60C until a constant weight was obtained. It was then cooled in a desiccator to yield dark-brown solid extract.

3.4. Phytochemical Evaluation

The crude extract was subjected to phytochemical screening using standard techniques of plant secondary metabolites. The extract was tested for alkaloid, flavournoids, saponins, tannins, Anthraquinoes, reducing sugar (in glycosides) catrdiac glycosides, and glycosides.

3.4.1. Test for Alkaloids

Test for alkaloids was performed using Wagner and Dragendoff reagents (Sofowora, 1994). 0.5g of the extract was added to 5ml of 1% aqueous hydrochloric acid on steam bath. This was filtered and 1ml portion treated with a few drops of Dragenddoff Reagent and another 1ml portion similarly treated with wagner's reagent. The formation of precipitates was an indication of the presence of alkaloids.

3.4.2. Test for Flavonoids (Sofowora, 1994)

Two grams of the sample was dissolved in water for 5mins and filtered. The filtrate was collected in a test tube; then, 5 drops of5% sodium hydroxide were added followed by addition of 2ml of 10% Hydrochloric acid. A yellow solution indicates the presence of flavonoids.

3.4.3. Test for Saponins (Sofowora, 1994)

One gram of the *hliotropium indicum linn* was boiled wit 10ml distilled water for 10 minutes and filtered whiles hot, then allowed to cool. 2.5ml of the filtrate was diluted with 10ml of distilled water and shaken vigorously and the two drops of castor oil were added to the solution and shaken vigorously for 2 minutes. Presence of frothing and stable emulsion indicate the presence of saponins.

3.4.4. test for Cardiac Glycosides (Trease and Evans 2002)

One gram of the powdered sample was boiled with 10ml of 80% alcohol for 5 minutes on a water bath filtered. The cooled filtrate was diluted with equal volume of distilled water and few drops of lead acetate was added and shaken thoroughly. This was allowed to stand for about 5 minutes and then filtered. The filtrate was extracted with 2 volumes of chloroform and the combined extracts were concentrated to form a residue that was used for Keller Killisni snd Kedde tests.

3.4.5. Keller-Killini`s Test:

A portion of chloroform extract was dissolved in ferric reagent (0.3ml of 10% ferric chloride in 50% glacial acetic acid) in clean test tubes. 2ml of concentrated sulphuric acid was carefully poured down the side of the test tube so as to form a layer below the acetic acid solution. The formation of purple, reddish brown or brown ring at the interphase and green colour in the acetic acid layer are characteristics of cardenolides. The test is used for the detection of 2-deoxy-sugar.

3.4.6. Kedde`s Test:

The second portion of the extract was mixed with 1ml of 3,5-dinitrobenzoic acid in ethanol. The resulting solution was made alkaline by adding 5% NaOH dropwise. The formation of brown purple colour indicates the presence of unsaturated lactone ring of sesquiterpenees.

3.4.7. test for Tannis (Trease and Evans, 2002)

About 0.5g of the powdered leaf samples was boiled with 10ml of distilled water for 5 minutes. It was filtered while hot and cooled. The filtrate was adjusted to 20ml with distilled water. An aliquot (1.0ml) of the filtrate was further diluted with distilled water to 5ml, after which a few drops of 0.1% ferric chloride solution were added. A bluish-black or greenish colour indicates a positive test.

3.4.8. Test for Anthraquinones

3.4.8.1. Combined the Anthraquinones

Half a gram of the powdered sample was boiled with 10mls of HCL (1%) for 5 minutes, filtered whilest hot and the filtrate allowed to cool. The cooled filtrate was then partitioned against equal volume of chloroform. The chloroform layer was carefully transferred into a clean test tube, shaken with an equal volume of 10% ammonia solution and the layer allowed to separate. The observation of a delicate rose pink colour indicates the presence of combined Anthraquinones (glycoside).

3.4.8.2 Free Anthraquinones

Half a gram of the powdered sample was placed in a dry test tube, 5ml of chloroform added and shaken for 5 minutes. The extracts were then filtered and filtrate shaken with equal volume of 10%

ammonia. The observation of a bright pink colour in the aqueous layer indicates presence of free Anthraquinones (aglycone).

3.4.9. Reducing sugar (in glycoside)

The extracts were dissolved to water and heated in water bath. Two milliter of the solution in a test tube was added to 1ml each of Fehling's solution A and B, the mixture was shaken heated in a water bath for 10 minutes A brick-red precipitate indicates the presence of reducing sugar.

3.4.10. Evaluation of anti-helminthic effect of Heliotropium indicum linn

Three different masses; 0.1500g,0.2000g and 0.2500g of the extracts were weighted into three different beakers and labelled. Each of the weighed extract in the beakers was mixed with 1 ml of distilled water; the mixture was shaken vigorously and allowed and stand for 5 minutes. One intestinal worm was then placed in the mixture and the time of the paralysis and time of death were taken and recorded. The test was done three time for each concentration and mean time of paralysis was determined.

3.4.11. Evaluation of Pesticidal effect of Heliotropium indicum linn

Three different masses; Three different masses; 0.1500g, 0.2000g and 0.2500g of the extracts were weighted into three different beakers and labelled. Each of the weighed extract in the beakers was mixed with 1 ml of distilled water; the mixture was shaken vigorously and allowed and stand for 5 minutes. One weevil was then placed in the mixture and it time of the paralysis and time of death were taken and recorded. The test was done three time for each concentration and mean time of death was determined.

3.4.12 Control Experiment

Distilled water was used as a control against helminthes and weevils.

3.4.12 Standard Drug

3.16.1. *Albendazole* was the standard drug used against helminthes.

3.16.2 *Actellic supper* was the standard drug used against weevil

CHAPTER FOUR: RESULTS

4.1 Phytochemical screening

Table 4.1: Flavonoids, Saponins, Tannins, and reducing sugars

	Flavonoid	Saponins	Tannins	Reducing sugar
Inflorescence	+	+	+	+
Leaves	+	+	+	+
Roots	+	-	-	+

Key: +, Means present and -, Means absent.

Phytochemical screening of the plant reveals the presence of flavonoids, saponins, tannins and reducing sugars for the inflorescences and leave extracts. However, the roots extract had only flavonoids, and reducing sugars present but saponins and tannins were absent.

Table 4.2: Alkaloids test using Wegner and Dragendorff reagents

	Wagner reagents	Dragendorff reagents
Inflorescence	+	+
Leaves	++	++
Roots	-	-

Key: +, Means present, ++, Means more present and -, Means absent.

From the table 4.2 above, alkaloids were present in the leaves extract more than the inflorescence extract but absent in the roots extract for both Wegner reagent and Dragendorff reagents.

Table 4.3: Anthraquines test

	Combine Anthraquines	Free Anthraquines
Inflorescence	+	-
Leaves	+	-
Roots	+	-

Key: +, Means present and -, Means absent.

Table 4.3: shows that combined Anthraquines was present in all the extracts and free Anthraquines was absent in all the extracts.

18

4.2 Effect of the plant extracts on helminthes

4.2.1 Mean time of paralysis

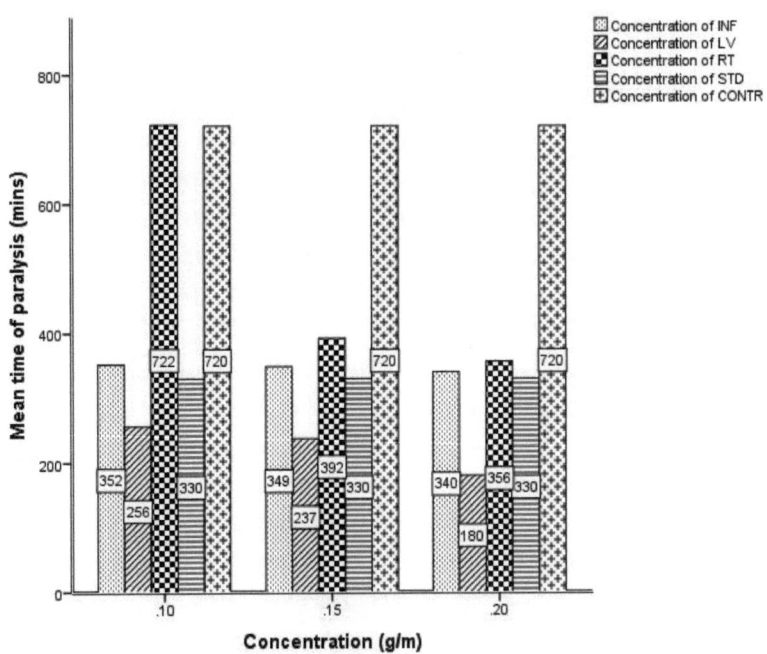

Figure 4.1: Mean time of paralysis of helminthes by the concentrations of extracts

From the Figure 4.1 above, the various concentrations of the plant extracts from inflorescence, leaves and root were able to paralyze the helminthes. The leave extract had faster mean time of paralysis than the inflorescence and the root extracts and even the standard drug. Followed by the inflorescence extract and then, the root extract, with the anti-helminthic effect increasing with increase in concentration of the extracts.

Table 4.8: Tests of Between-Subjects Effects – Helminthic (mean time of paralysis)

Source	Dependent Variable	Type III Sum of Squares	df	Mean Square	F	p-value
Corrected Model	0.10	388377.067[a]	4	97094.267	6711.585	.000
	0.15	409131.600[b]	4	102282.900	21308.938	.000
	0.20	480012.267[c]	4	120003.067	22785.392	.000
Within concentrations	0.10	388377.067	4	97094.267	6711.585	.000
	0.15	409131.600	4	102282.900	21308.937	.000
	0.20	480012.267	4	120003.067	22785.392	.000

Multivariate two-way analysis of variance (MANOVA) was conducted to measure the significant differences of the mean time of paralysis between and within concentrations. Using the Turkey post hoc analysis test, *Test of Between-Subject Effect* was determined to measure whether significant difference exist (i.e. p-value <0.05) for the mean time of paralysis of helminthes under different concentration as presented in the table above. From the results, p-value <0.05 between and within concentrations, which indicates that significant differences exist for the mean time of paralysis effect of the extracts on helminthes under different concentration.

4.2.2 Mean time of death

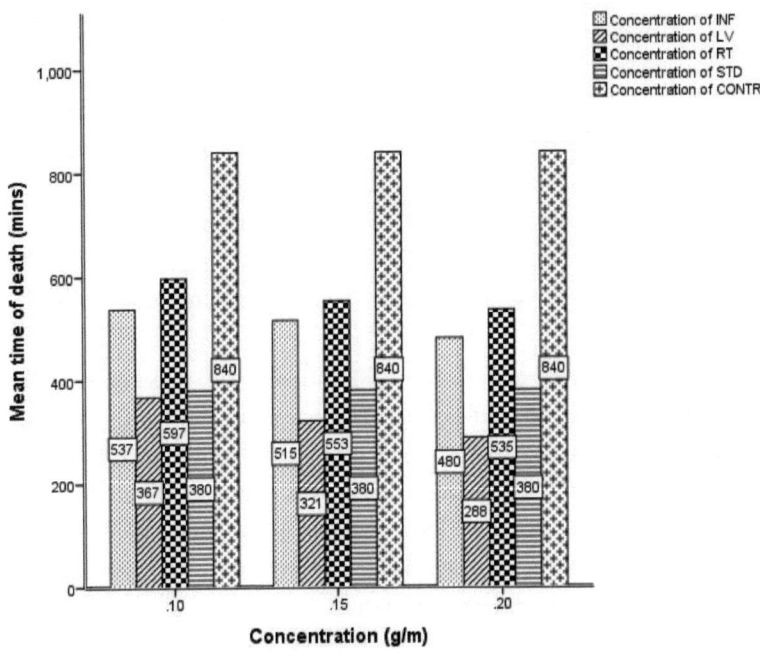

Figure 4.2: Mean time of death of helminthes by the concentrations of extracts

From the Figure 4.2 above, the various concentrations of the plant extracts from inflorescence, leaves and root were able to kill the helminthes. The leave extract had faster mean time of death than the inflorescence and the root extracts and even the standard drug. Followed by the inflorescence extract and then, the root extract, with the anti-helminthic effect increasing with increase in concentration of the extracts.

Table 4.10: Tests of Between-Subjects Effects – Helminthic (mean time of death)

Source	Dependent Variable	Type III Sum of Squares	df	Mean Square	F	p-value
Corrected Model	0.10	443699.600[a]	4	110924.900	9963.314	.000
	0.15	487342.933[b]	4	121835.733	16031.018	.000
	0.20	529450.667[c]	4	132362.667	10129.796	.000
Within concentrations	0.10	443699.600	4	110924.900	9963.314	.000
	0.15	487342.933	4	121835.733	16031.018	.000
	0.20	529450.667	4	132362.667	10129.796	.000

Multivariate two-way analysis of variance (MANOVA) was conducted to measure the significant differences of the mean time of death between and within concentrations. Using the Turkey post hoc analysis test, *Test of Between-Subject Effect* was determined to measure whether significant difference exist (i.e. p-value <0.05) for the mean time of death under different concentrations of the extracts as presented in the table above. From the results, p-value <0.05 between and within concentrations, which indicates that significant differences exist for the mean time of death effect of the extracts on helminthes under different concentration.

4.3 Effect of the plant extracts on weevil

4.3.1 Mean time of paralysis

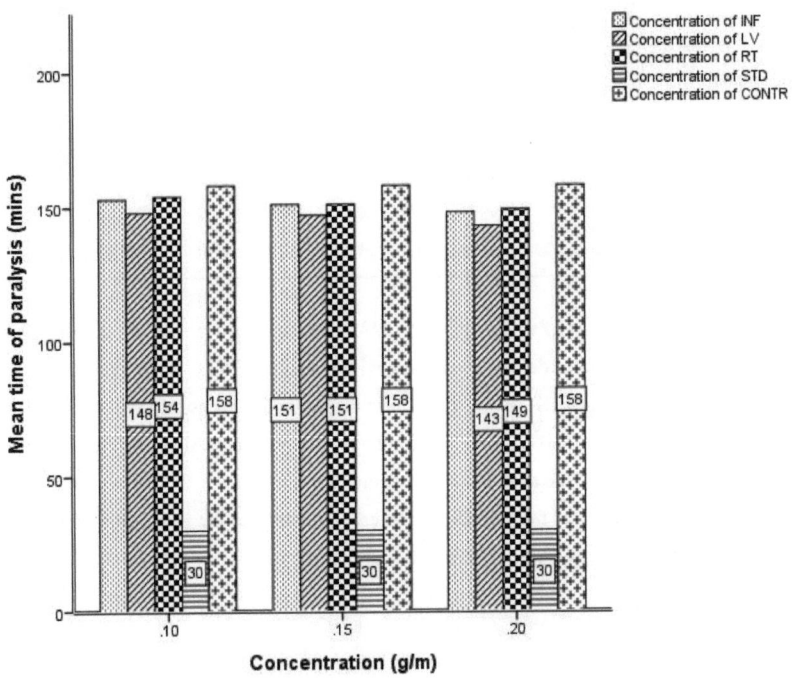

Figure 4.3: Mean time of paralysis of weevil by the concentrations of extracts

From the Figure 4.3 above, the leave extract showed a shorter mean time of paralysis than the other extracts. The mean time of paralysis of the inflorescence and the root extracts were almost the same, both extract had very little effect on the weevil. But the standard paralyzed the weevil far faster than all the extracts.

Table 4.15: Tests of Between-Subjects Effects – Weevil (mean time of paralysis)

Source	Dependent Variable	Type III Sum of Squares	df	Mean Square	F	p-value
Corrected Model	0.10	36600.267[a]	4	9150.067	473.279	.000
	0.15	35811.067[b]	4	8952.767	495.541	.000
	0.20	34766.400[c]	4	8691.600	472.370	.000
Within Concentrations	0.10	36600.267	4	9150.067	473.279	.000
	0.15	35811.067	4	8952.767	495.541	.000
	0.20	34766.400	4	8691.600	472.370	.000

Multivariate two-way analysis of variance (MANOVA) was conducted to measure the significant differences of the mean time of death between and within concentrations. Using the Turkey post hoc analysis test, *Test of Between-Subject Effect* was determined to measure whether significant difference exist (i.e. p-value <0.05) for the mean time of paralysis under different concentrations of the extracts as presented in the table above. From the results, p-value <0.05 between and within concentrations, which indicates that significant differences exist for the mean time of paralysis effect of the extracts on weevil under different concentration.

4.3.2 Mean time of death

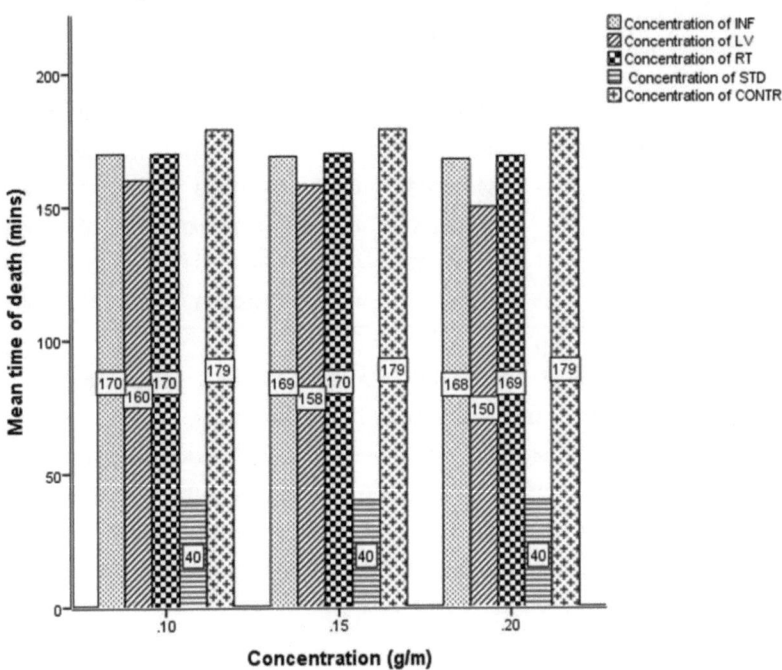

Figure 4.4: Mean time of paralysis of weevil by the concentrations of extracts

From the Figure 4.4 above, the leave extract showed a shorter mean time of paralysis than the other extracts. The mean time of paralysis of the inflorescence and the root extracts were almost the same, both extract had very little effect on the weevil. But the standard paralyzed the weevil far faster than all the extracts.

Table 4.17: Tests of Between-Subjects Effects – Weevil (mean time of death)

Source	Dependent Variable	Type III Sum of Squares	df	Mean Square	F	p-value
Corrected Model	0.10	41084.000[a]	4	10271.000	723.310	.000
	0.15	40529.733[b]	4	10132.433	1369.248	.000
	0.20	39608.933[c]	4	9902.233	934.173	.000
Within Concentrations	0.10	41084.000	4	10271.000	723.310	.000
	0.15	40529.733	4	10132.433	1369.248	.000
	0.20	39608.933	4	9902.233	934.173	.000

Multivariate two-way analysis of variance (MANOVA) was conducted to measure the significant differences of the mean time of death between and within concentrations. Using the Turkey post hoc analysis test, *Test of Between-Subject Effect* was determined to measure whether significant difference exist (i.e. p-value <0.05) for the mean time of death under different concentrations of the extracts as presented in the table above. From the results, p-value <0.05 between and within concentrations, which indicates that significant differences exist for the mean time of death effect of the extracts on weevil under different concentration.

CHAPTER FIVE: DISCUSSION, CONCLUTION AND RECOMMENDATION

5.1. Phytochemical screening

Phytochemical screening of extracts showed the presence of flavonoid, saponins, tannins, reducing sugars, alkaloid and combined Anthraquinones. But saponins, tannins, and alkaloid were absent in the root extract. Free Anthraquinones was absent in all the extracts. The detection of saponin and tannins in the aqueous extract of *helotropium indicum* supports the earlier reports of Alkinlolu *et al.* (2008). However, observation in this study further revealed the presence of alkaloids in the aqueous extract of *heliotropium indicum* as said by Adeleja *et al,* (2008).

5.2. Evaluation of anti-helminthic effect of *Heliotropium indicum linn*

Figure 4.1 and figure 4.2 clearly revealed that leaves extract have very high anti-helminthic properties than the inflorescence and the root extracts and even the standard drug, followed by the inflorescence and then, the roots with the effect increasing with increase in concentration of the

26

extracts (Statistically, there was significant difference within each concentration and between the concentrations for the extracts). However, the standard shows more anti-helminthic activity or property than the root extract. This anti-helminthic activity or property observed may be attributed to these phytochemicals; Flavonoids, Saponins, Tannins and Alkaloids.

This work therefore corroborates the finding by Adelaja et al. (2008) who reported the histo-gastroprotective of this plant extract on laboratory winster rats and linked the observed results to the presence of saponins, tannins and alkaloids in *Heliotrapium indicum*. The low anti-helminthic properties of the roots extract may be as a result of the absence of some phytochemicals, alkaloid, saponins and tannins in the extract or the inability of the solvent to extract the phytochemicals in the roots. Probably, the high potency of the leaves and inflorescence extracts might be due to the alkaloid content or combination of other components that are absent in the root extracts (Abdulazeez *et al,* 2005). The leaves extract potency may be due to the high level of alkaloid present.

5.3. Evaluation of pesticidal effect of *Heliotropium linn*

The results from figure 4.3 and 4.4 showed that there is not any much effect of the extracts on the weevil as compared to the standard drug. Using turkey HSD Multiple comparison there was a significant difference between the means time of the standard drug and the extracts (i,e. p-value <0.05), there was no significant difference between the mean time of the extracts for the 0.10g/ml concentration, and also no significant difference between the meant time of the control between the inflorescence, and the root difference, except the leave.

The standard chemical from figure 4.3. and 4.4 shows very high pesticidal effect far than all the extracts with about 2-hour time intervals. This low potency or low pesticidal effect may be attributed to the exoskeleton of the weevil, which makes it difficult for the extract to penetrate and denature the organism. Since these extracts are highly potent on the helminth which has very delicate or soft exoskeleton, it is hypothesized that the exoskeleton of the weevil hindered the penetration of the extracts and in effect reduced their effect on the organism (lzzo *et al,* 2011).

5.4. CONCLUTION

The mean time/hrs of paralysis for helminthes were (5:52, 5:49, and 5:40), (4:16, 3:57, and 3:00) and (7:02, 6:56) for (0.1g/ml, 0.15g/ml and 0.2g/ml) concentrations for inflorescence, leaves, and roots extracts respectively. And the mean time/hrs of paralysis from weevils were (2:33, 2:31 and 2:28), (2:28, 2:27 and 2:23) and (2:24, 2:21 and 2:30) for (0.1g/ml, 0.15g/ml and 0.2g/ml) for

27

inflorescence, leaves and roots extracts respectively. And mean time of death for helminthes were (8:57, 8:35, and 8:00), (6:07, 5:21, and 4:48) and 9:57, 9:13, and 8:55) for (0.1g/ml, 0.15g/ml and 0.2g/ml) concentrations for inflorescence, leaves, and roots extracts respectively. And the mean time/hrs of death for weevils were (2:50, 2:49 and 2:48), (2:40, 2:38 and 2:30) and (2:50, 2:50 and 2:49) for (0.1g/ml, 0.15g/ml and 0.2g/ml) concentrations for inflorescence, leaves, and roots extracts respectively.

The results revealed that the leaves extract < inflorescence extract < root extract have significant anti-helminthic property but no or in significant pesticide property.

5.5. RECOMMENDATION

It is recommended that the extracts should be tried on the larva of a weevil before applying on the organism to compare the effects.

Also advance study can be conducted on the leave or a combination of extracts from the various parts of the plants to support their effect and purification of the plant and toxicological examination towards its adoption as a deworming drug for poultry or animals or humans.

REFERENCES

Abeloff, A. (2008). Abeloff's Clinical Oncology, 4th ed. Pheladelphia, P. A. Churchill Livingstone, an Imprint of Elsevier

Ainsle, J. R. (1937). Lists of plants used in Native Medicine in Nigeria, sp. No. 177. Oxford University.

Altschuler, J. A., Casella, S. J., MacKenzie, T. A and Curtis, K. M. (2007). The effect of cinnamom on AIC among adolescents with type 1 diabetes. Diabetes Care, 813-816

Backstorm-Sternber, SM, Duke A (1994). Potential for synergistic action of phytochemical in spice. Spices, herbs and edible fungi, Cheralambous, G. (Ed.), Elsevier Science, B. V., New York, USA, page 201-223

Moquin, B., Marc, R., Blackman, M. D., Mitty, E and Flores, S. (2009). Complementary and alternative medicine (CAM), Vol. 30, Issue 3, 196-203

Bhikha, R. A.H., Mohamed, N. (2004). The little book of Tibb. Johannesburg, IBN Sina Institute of Tibb.

Bhikha, R. A. H and Haq, M. A (2000). Tibb-traditional roots of medicine in modern routes to health. South Africa. Performance? *Psychology Bulletin*, Vol 121, p. 171-191.

Boivin, M. J. and Giordiani, B. (1993). Improvements in cognitive performance for school children in Zaire, Africa: Following an iron supplement and treatment for intestinal parasite. *Journal of Paediatric Psychology*, Vol. 18. P. 249-264.

Borkow, G. and Bentwich, Z. (2000). Eradication of helminthic infection may be essential for successful vaccination against HIV and tuberculosis. *Bulletin of the World Health Organization*, Vol. 78.

Bradstrrt, K. (1997). *Herbs for detoxification,* Woodland Publications

Burkill, I. H. (1935). A dictionary of the economic products of Malay Peninsula. Edited by: Ministry of Agriculture (Malaysia). Crown Agents for Colonies. London, p. 1136.

Chaudhurry, R. R. (1992). Herbal Medicine for human health, WHO (SEARO, No. 20), Chinese Statistical Bureau, Beijn, China.

Crompton, D. W. T. (1992). Human nutrition and parasitic infection. Cambridge University Press.

Dalziel, J. M. (1937). The useful plant of West Africa. Royal Botanic Gardens, p. 64-69.

Damery, S., Gratus, C., Grieve, R., et al. (2011). The use of herbal medicine by people with cancer: a cross-sectional survey. *Br. J. Cancer*, p. 927-933.

29

Dans, A. M., Villarruz, M. V. Jimeno, C. A., et al. (2007). The effect of momordica charantia capsule preparation on glycemic control in type 2 diabetics mellitus needs further studies. *Journal of Clinical Epidemiology, p. 554-559.*

Moher, D., Soeken, K., Sampson, M., Bem-Porat, L., and Berman, B. (2008). Assessing the quality of reports of systematic reviews in paediatric complementary and alternative medicine, vol. 2.

Rosso, D., Miller, J., and Marek, T. (1996). Class action: improving school performance in developing world through better health and nutrition. The World Bank, Direction in Development.

Dos Santos-Neto, L. L., de Vilhena-Toledo, M. A., Medeiros-Souza, P and de Souza, G. A. (2006). The use of herbal medicine in Alzhemeir's disease – a systematic review. *Evidence based Complement Alternative Medicine,* p. 441-445.

Swisher, M. E., Cohn, E. D., Goff, A. B., Parham, J., Herzog, J. T., Rader, S. J and Mutch, G. D. (2002). Use of complementary and alternative medicine among women with gynaecologic cancers, Vol. 84, Issue 3, p. 363-367.

Ezeamama, A. E. (2005). Helminth infection and cognitive impairment among Filipino Children. *The American Journal of Tropical Medical Hygiene, Vol. 72, p. 540-548.*

Environmental Protection Agency (EPA), (Thursday 29, 2009). Types of pesticides.

FEPA, (19929). Country study report for Nigeria on cost-benefits and unmet needs of biological diversity conservation.

Food and Agricultural Organization of the United State, (2009). International Code of Conduct on the distribution and use of pesticides.

Koffuor, G. A., Boy, A., Ameyaw, E. O., Amoateng, P and Abaitey, A., (2012). Hypothesis effect of aqueous extract of *Heliotropium indicumn Linn (Boraginaceae)*

Gilbert, B. Ferreira, J. L. P., Almeida, M. B. S., Carvalho, E. S., Cascon, V., Rocha, L. M., (1997). The official use of medicinal plants in public health. Journal of the Brazilian Association for Advancement of Science 49, page 339-334.

Gratus, C, Wilson, S., Greenfield, S. M., Damery, S. L., Warmington, S. A., Grieve, R., Steven, N. M., Routledge, P., (May, 2009). The use of herbal medicines by people with cancer: a qualitative study. *Complement Alternative Medicine.*

Hammond-Tooke, D., (1989). Rituals and medicines: Indigenous healing in South Africa. A, D, Donker. Johannesburg.

Hansan, S. S., Ahmed, S. I., Bukhari, N. I., London, W. C., (Aug. 2009). Use of complementary and alternative medicine among patients with chronic diseases at outpatient clinics. *Complement The Clinic Practice, page 152-157.*

Irvine, J. R., (1961). Woody Plants of Ghana, Second Edition, London, Oxford University Press. Page 58.

Izzo A. A., Ernest E., (2011). Interactions between herbal medicines and prescription drugs: an updated systematic review. Drugs, page 1777-1798

John, D. T., William, A. and Petri, J., (2006). *Markell and Vogue's Medical Parasitology, 9th Edition.* Saunders Elsevier Press.

Osemene, K. P., Elujoba, A. A., and Hori, M. O., (2011). A Comparative Assessment of Herbal and Orthodox Medicines in Nigeria. *Research Journal of Medical Sciences, Vol. 5, Issue 5, page 280-285.*

APPENDIX

4.4: Evaluation of anti-helminthic effect of the influences (INF) extract

Concentration	Time of Paralysis (hrs)				Time of death (hrs)			
(g/ml)	Tp1	Tp2	Tp3	MTp	Td1	Td2	Td3	MTd
0.10g in 1mil	5:49	5:57	5:52	**5:52**	8:52	8:57	9:02	**8:57**
0.15g in 1ml	5:51	5:49	5:47	**5:49**	8:35	8:32	8:39	**8:35**
0.20g in 1mil	5:40	5:39	5:41	**5:40**	8:07	7:58	7:55	**8:00**

KEY: Tp means time of paralysis, Td means time of death, MTp means mean time of paralysis and MTd means mean time of death.

4.5: Evaluation of anti-helminthic effect of the leaves (LV) extract

Concentration	Time of Paralysis (hrs)				Time of death (hrs)			
(g/ml)	Tp1	Tp2	Tp3	MTp	Td1	Td2	Td3	MTd
0.10g in 1mil	4:15	4:22	4:11	**4:16**	6:02	6:07	6:11	**6:07**
0.15g in 1ml	3:54	3:58	3:59	**3:57**	5:19	5:25	5:21	**5:21**
0.20g in 1mil	2:56	3:04	3:01	**3:00**	4:45	4:51	4:48	**4:48**

4.6: Evaluation of anti-helminthic effect of the roots (RT) extract.

Concentration	Time of Paralysis (hrs)				Time of death (hrs)			
(g/ml)	Tp1	Tp2	Tp3	MTp	Td1	Td2	Td3	MTd
0.10g in 1mil	6:57	7:07	7:02	**7:02**	9:49	9:44	9:50	**9:57**
0.15g in 1ml	6:36	6:31	6:29	**6:32**	9:14	9:09	9:17	**9:13**
0.20g in 1mil	5:56	5:53	5:59	**5:56**	8:52	8:54	9:00	**8:55**

Table 4.7: Descriptive statistics – Helminthic (mean time of paralysis)

Concentrations		Mean (mins)	Std. Deviation	N
	CONT	720.0000[e]	.00000	3
	INF	352.6667[c]	4.04145	3
0.10g in 1ml	LV	256.0000[a]	5.56776	3
	RT	422.0000[d]	5.00000	3
	STD	330.0000[b]	.00000	3
0.15g in 1ml	CONT	720.0000[e]	.00000	3

32

	INF	349.0000[c]	2.00000	3
	LV	237.0000[a]	2.64575	3
	RT	392.0000[d]	3.60555	3
	STD	330.0000[b]	.00000	3
	CONT	720.0000[e]	.00000	3
	INF	340.0000[c]	1.00000	3
0.20g in 1ml	LV	180.3333[a]	4.04145	3
	RT	356.0000[d]	3.00000	3
	STD	330.0000[b]	.00000	3

Table 4.9: Descriptive statistics – Helminthic (mean time of death)

Concentrations		Mean (mins)	Std. Deviation	N
	CONT	840.0000[e]	.00000	3
	INF	537.0000[c]	5.00000	3
0.10g in 1ml	LV	366.6667[a]	4.50925	3
	RT	587.6667[d]	3.21455	3
	STD	380.0000[b]	.00000	3
	CONT	840.0000[e]	.00000	3
	INF	515.3333[c]	3.51188	3
0.15g in 1ml	LV	321.6667[a]	3.05505	3
	RT	553.3333[d]	4.04145	3
	STD	380.0000[b]	.00000	3
	CONT	840.0000[e]	.00000	3
	INF	480.0000[c]	6.24500	3
0.20g in 1ml	LV	288.0000[a]	3.00000	3
	RT	535.3333[d]	4.16333	3
	STD	380.0000[b]	.00000	3

4.11: Evaluation of pesticidal effect of the influences (INF) extract using weevil

Concentration	Time of Paralysis (hrs)				Time of death (hrs)			
(g/ml)	Tp1	Tp2	Tp3	MTp	Td1	Td2	Td3	MTd
0.10g in 1mil	2:32	2:29	2:37	**2:33**	2:49	2:51	2:51	**2:50**

0.15g in 1ml	2:29	2:26	2:36	**2:31**	2:52	2:47	2:47	**2:49**
0.20g in 1mil	2:20	2:27	2:37	**2:28**	2:46	2:48	2:49	**2:48**

KEY: Tp means time of paralysis, Td means time of death, MTp means mean time of paralysis and MTd means mean time of death.

4.12: Evaluation of pesticidal effect of the leaves (LV) extract using weevil

Concentration	Time of Paralysis (hrs)				Time of death (hrs)			
(g/ml)	Tp1	Tp2	Tp3	MTp	Td1	Td2	Td3	MTd
0.10g in 1mil	2:24	2:32	2:29	**2:28**	2:39	2:45	2:37	**2:40**
0.15g in 1ml	2:22	2:33	2:26	**2:27**	2:37	2:38	2:40	**2:33**
0.20g in 1mil	2:19	2:25	2:25	**2:23**	2:22	2:29	2:32	**2:30**

4.13: Evaluation of peticidal effect of the roots (RT) extract using weevil

Concentration	Time of Paralysis (hrs)				Time of death (hrs)			
(g/ml)	Tp1	Tp2	Tp3	MTp	Td1	Td2	Td3	MTd
0.10g in 1mil	2:34	2:26	2:42	**2:34**	2:42	2:55	2:54	**2:50**
0.15g in 1ml	2:32	2:24	2:37	**2:31**	2:54	2:51	2:44	**2:50**
0.20g in 1mil	2:28	2:33	2:29	**2:29**	2:46	2:47	2:55	**2:49**

Table 4.14: Descriptive statistics – Weevil (mean time of paralysis)

Concentration		Mean	Std. Deviation	N
	CONT	158.0000	.00000	3
	INF	152.6667	4.04145	3
0.10g in 1ml	LV	148.3333	4.04145	3
	RT	154.0000	8.00000	3
	STD	30.0000	.00000	3
	CONT	158.0000	.00000	3
	INF	151.3333	4.04145	3
0.15g in 1ml	LV	147.0000	5.56776	3
	RT	151.0000	6.55744	3
	STD	30.0000	.00000	3

	CONT	158.0000	.00000	3
	INF	148.0000	8.54400	3
0.20g in 1ml	LV	143.0000	3.46410	3
	RT	150.0000	2.64575	3
	STD	30.0000	.00000	3

Table 4.16: Descriptive statistics – Weevil (mean time of death)

Concentration		Mean	Std. Deviation	N
	CONT	179.0000	.00000	3
	INF	170.3333	1.15470	3
0.10g in 1ml	LV	160.3333	4.16333	3
	RT	170.3333	7.23418	3
	STD	40.0000	.00000	3
	CONT	179.0000	.00000	3
	INF	168.6667	2.88675	3
0.15g in 1ml	LV	158.3333	1.52753	3
	RT	169.6667	5.13160	3
	STD	40.0000	.00000	3
	CONT	179.0000	.00000	3
	INF	167.6667	1.52753	3
0.20g in 1ml	LV	147.6667	5.13160	3
	RT	169.3333	4.93288	3
	STD	40.0000	.00000	3

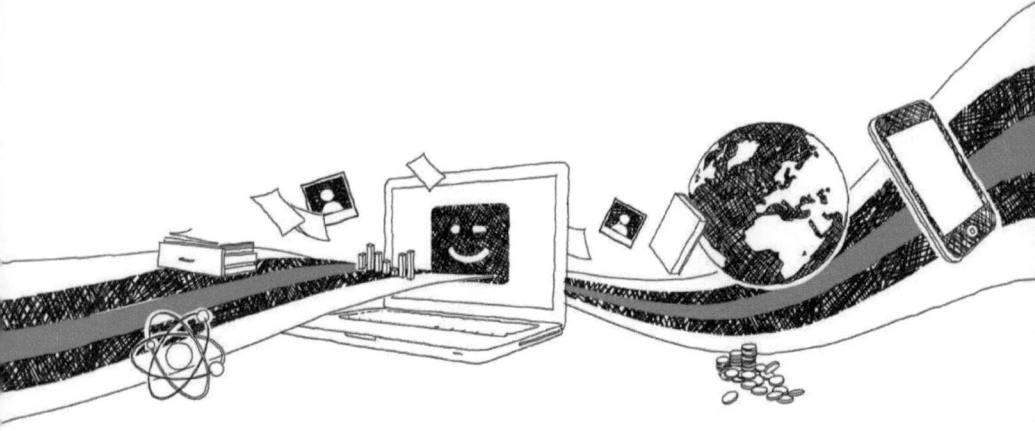
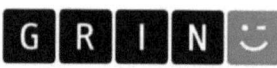